The **RESTART** Journal

A three-month daily journal to track your progress and make connections between the food you eat, the habits you keep, and the way you feel.

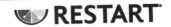

If you haven't taken The RESTART® Program, here's a bit of information about it...

RESTART® Your Health In Just 5 Weeks!

What is the RESTART® Program? It is part nutritional class, part sugar detox, and part support group - a powerful and empowering set up for success.

The RESTART® Program is a simple, powerful way to give your body a vacation from sugar and processed foods. With a 3-week sugar detox built right in, the program focuses on how to use REAL FOOD to boost your energy, reduce inflammation and get rid of sugar and carb cravings. You will discover how good you can feel!

REAL FOOD, REAL LEARNING, REAL SUPPORT = *real results!*

 # TAKE THE CLASS

Are you ready to RESTART?
To find classes in your area or online, visit www.TheRestartProgram.com and click on FIND A CLASS.

An introduction from the creator of The RESTART® Program

In RESTART® we understand the power of real food - how it can support us or hinder us. We don't "count" things like calories or macros. Instead, we tune into our body. Often we don't realize what our own bodies are telling us.

I hope you will use this journal to tune into the messages your body has for you.

Remember, this is YOUR journal. No one is judging it. Stay open and curious to what you discover.

If you are working with a holistic nutrition practitioner, this journal will become instrumental in your healing journey, but remember, the most important person to know what goes in here is you.

You've got this!

Jeni

Jeni Hall, NTP
Creator of The RESTART® Program

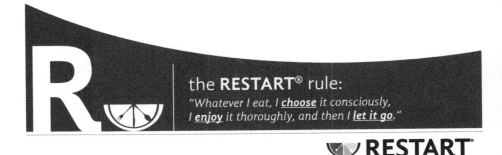

the **RESTART®** rule:
*"Whatever I eat, I **choose** it consciously, I **enjoy** it thoroughly, and then I **let it go**."*

RESTART

You are holding a powerful tool of self-discovery.

This journal will help you to be more in tune with your body. By consciously paying attention to what and how often you eat and drink, how much or how little you move your body, how you sleep, and how you feel in response to these things, it will provide you with important clues. You will begin to connect the dots between diet and lifestyle and what your body wants and needs to function at its best.

Use this powerful tool to help you connect to yourself.

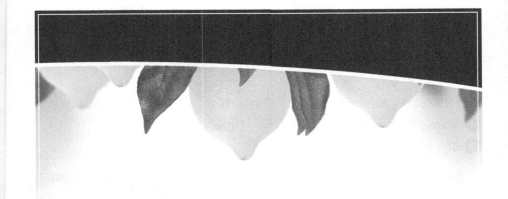

HOW TO USE
your journal...

1 **Today is:** ....

2 **Yesterday's bedtime:**   :   **Woke up at:**   :   **3** **Sleep quality:**

4 **Water:** ☐☐☐☐☐☐☐☐☐☐ (10 oz or 296 ml per box)

5 **BM:** ☐ Yes ☐ No   **BSC #:**

Time	What I Ate & Drank	How I Feel
	6	

HOW TO USE THIS JOURNAL - left hand page

There are plenty of cues and suggestions that will guide your journaling activity, but ultimately the choice is yours. Use this tool in a way that makes the most sense to you.

1 **"Today is"** - This can be a calendar date, or day of the week. If you are using the journal during the 21 days of The RESTART® Program, you could record numbers 1 through 21 here if you choose.

2 **"Yesterday's bedtime"** - Record when you went to bed and when you woke up.

3 **"Sleep quality"**- was it restful? Restless? Not long enough? You can write a word to describe it, or use a scale of 1-5 and rate it... If you want to note more about your sleep, you can add your observations to your daily Reflections.

4 **"Water"** - This is a priority! How much water should you drink? A simple formula is to divide your weight in half and drink that many ounces of water. For example, if you weigh 150 lbs, strive to drink 75 ounces of plain water per day (150 ÷ 2 = 75). Don't forget to listen to your body. Your needs may vary with activity levels, climate, or other factors. (Up to maximum of 100 ounces.)

5 **"BM"** - Bowel Movements. Did you have any? Yes or No. Hopefully your answer is yes, at least one BM per day is optimal.

Refer to the Bristol Stool Chart from the Digestion lesson in The RESTART® Program to determine your BSC # (you can use a search engine to find this chart online as well).

6 **Food record** - Record your daily eating details. Don't leave anything out. There is no judgment here. All information is useful. The "How I Feel" column is for you to notice how you feel before and/ or after your meals or snacks. It could be a physical sensation, like satiated, still hungry, sleepy, bloated, good energy, etc. or more of an emotional response, like irritable, content, focused, etc. If you want to note more about how you feel, you can add your observations to your daily Reflections.

Noting these responses can be an eye opener. Do you discover that you snack or "graze" all day? Do you forget (or are you too busy) to eat or drink? Do you discover that certain foods trigger symptoms? How does your energy level change throughout the day? All of these observations can help you understand where adjustments in foods and eating habits can help you feel and function at your best.

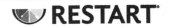 **RESTART**

HOW TO USE THIS JOURNAL - right hand page

(7) **"Today's Physical Activity"** – How did you move your body today? Also think about the time you spend just sitting. If it's time to get moving, choose something you know you will enjoy, so you will look forward to it.

(8) **"Today's good habit"** – What healthy habit are you working on today? This can be the same habit each day until you have mastered it, or you can add something new to work on and keep the challenge fresh. We've included a handy chart at the back of this journal to help you track your progress.

(9) **"Today I loved my body by"** - This is to remind you that self-care is so important! Take some time each day to give your body some love! It can be remembering to breathe deeply, or focus on good posture. It can be taking a relaxing bath, enjoying a foot massage, or reading a great book. It can be saying "No" or "Yes" to something. Don't forget positive affirmations and gratitude. There are so many ways to love your body – you deserve it!

(10) **"Reflections"** – you have a whole page each day to make your own observations about whatever you want. What are you learning about yourself? How do you feel about this process? Are you noticing changes? Are you making connections between food, activity, habits and how you feel?

A journey toward better health begins by knowing yourself.

Reflections:

7 Today's physical activity: ....

8 Today's good habit: ....

....

9 ♡ Today I loved my body by: ....

10

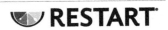 RESTART

MAKING
connections...

After you've been using your RESTART® Journal for a while, you will begin to see direct connections between food and specific responses in your body.

This information is incredibly important. Symptoms such as poor digestion, irritability, congestion, interrupted sleep, low energy and even aches and pains can seem like they're just "normal" parts of life or passed off as part of the aging process.

You may be surprised to realize that you could be feeling one or more of those things because of something that you regularly eat. A food might be "healthy" but if YOUR body doesn't respond well to it, none of that matters.

By noting the response you have to specific foods, you can make the best choices for your health and body.

You will also notice direct correlations between daily habits and how you feel. For example, if you move your body regularly, you may notice better sleep. If you drink more water, you may notice more energy or easier elimination, etc.

What connections are you making?

When I...	I notice I feel...

Examples: When I eat bread, I notice that I feel irritable and tired.

When I drink more water, I notice that I feel more energized and my skin is softer.

When I...	I notice I feel...

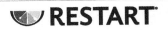

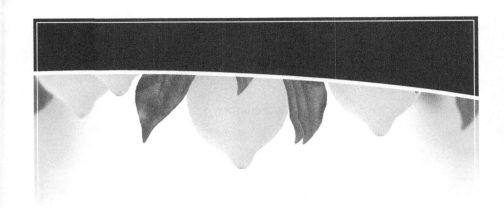

The **RESTART®** Journal
let's get started...

Today is:

Yesterday's bedtime: ___:___   Woke up at: ___:___   Sleep quality:

Water: ☐☐☐☐☐☐☐☐☐☐ (10 oz or 296 ml per box)

BM: ☐ Yes ☐ No   BSC #:

Time	What I Ate & Drank	How I Feel

Reflections:

Today's physical activity: ....

Today's good habit: ....

♡ **Today I loved my body by:** ....

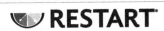

Today is:

Yesterday's bedtime: : Woke up at: : Sleep quality:

Water: ☐☐☐☐☐☐☐☐☐☐ (10 oz or 296 ml per box)

BM: ☐ Yes ☐ No BSC #:

Time	What I Ate & Drank	How I Feel

DAILY JOURNAL

Reflections:

Today's physical activity: ....

Today's good habit: ....

♡ **Today I loved my body by:** ....

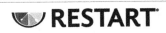

Today is:

Yesterday's bedtime: :   Woke up at: :   Sleep quality:

Water: ☐☐☐☐☐☐☐☐☐☐ (10 oz or 296 ml per box)

BM: ☐ Yes ☐ No   BSC #:

Time	What I Ate & Drank	How I Feel

DAILY JOURNAL

Reflections:

Today's physical activity: ....

Today's good habit: ....

....

♡ **Today I loved my body by:** ....

....

....

....

....

....

....

....

....

....

....

....

....

....

....

....

....

....

....

....

....

....

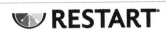

Today is:

Yesterday's bedtime: : Woke up at: : Sleep quality:

Water: ☐☐☐☐☐☐☐☐☐ (10 oz or 296 ml per box)

BM: ☐ Yes ☐ No BSC #:

Time	What I Ate & Drank	How I Feel

Reflections:

Today's physical activity: ....

Today's good habit: ....

♡ **Today I loved my body by:** ....

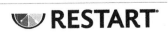

Today is:

Yesterday's bedtime: :   Woke up at: :   Sleep quality:

Water: ☐☐☐☐☐☐☐☐☐ (10 oz or 296 ml per box)

BM: ☐ Yes   ☐ No   BSC #:

Time	What I Ate & Drank	How I Feel

Reflections:

Today's physical activity: ....

Today's good habit: ....

....

♡ **Today I loved my body by:** ....

....

....

....

....

....

....

....

....

....

....

....

....

....

....

....

....

....

....

....

....

....

....

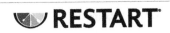

Today is:

Yesterday's bedtime: :   Woke up at: :   Sleep quality:

Water: ☐☐☐☐☐☐☐☐☐☐ (10 oz or 296 ml per box)

BM: ☐ Yes   ☐ No   BSC #:

Time	What I Ate & Drank	How I Feel

Reflections:

Today's physical activity: ....

Today's good habit: ....

♡ **Today I loved my body by:** ....

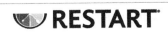

Today is:

Yesterday's bedtime: :   Woke up at: :   Sleep quality:

Water: ☐☐☐☐☐☐☐☐☐☐ (10 oz or 296 ml per box)

BM: ☐ Yes ☐ No   BSC #:

Time	What I Ate & Drank	How I Feel

Reflections:

Today's physical activity: ....

Today's good habit: ....

....

♡ **Today I loved my body by:** ....

....

....

....

....

....

....

....

....

....

....

....

....

....

....

....

....

....

....

....

....

....

....

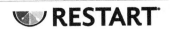

Today is:

Yesterday's bedtime: :   Woke up at: :   Sleep quality:

Water: ☐☐☐☐☐☐☐☐☐ (10 oz or 296 ml per box)

BM: ☐ Yes   ☐ No   BSC #:

Time	What I Ate & Drank	How I Feel

DAILY JOURNAL

Reflections:

Today's physical activity: ....

Today's good habit: ....

♡ Today I loved my body by: ....

....

....

....

....

....

....

....

....

....

....

....

....

....

....

....

....

....

....

....

....

....

....

....

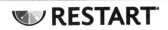

Today is:

Yesterday's bedtime: :   Woke up at: :   Sleep quality:

Water: ☐☐☐☐☐☐☐☐☐ (10 oz or 296 ml per box)

BM: ☐ Yes   ☐ No   BSC #:

Time	What I Ate & Drank	How I Feel

DAILY JOURNAL

Reflections:

Today's physical activity: ....

Today's good habit: ....

♡ **Today I loved my body by:** ....

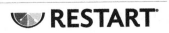

Today is:

Yesterday's bedtime: : Woke up at: : Sleep quality:

Water: ☐☐☐☐☐☐☐☐☐ (10 oz or 296 ml per box)

BM: ☐ Yes ☐ No BSC #:

Time	What I Ate & Drank	How I Feel

Reflections:

Today's physical activity: ....

Today's good habit: ....

♡ **Today I loved my body by:** ....

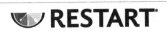

Today is:

Yesterday's bedtime: :   Woke up at: :   Sleep quality:

Water: ☐☐☐☐☐☐☐☐☐ (10 oz or 296 ml per box)

BM: ☐ Yes   ☐ No   BSC #:

Time	What I Ate & Drank	How I Feel

Reflections:

Today's physical activity: ....

Today's good habit: ....

....

♡ **Today I loved my body by:** ....

....

....

....

....

....

....

....

....

....

....

....

....

....

....

....

....

....

....

....

....

....

....

....

....

....

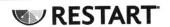

Today is:

Yesterday's bedtime: :   Woke up at: :   Sleep quality:

Water: ☐ ☐ ☐ ☐ ☐ ☐ ☐ ☐ ☐ (10 oz or 296 ml per box)

BM: ☐ Yes   ☐ No   BSC #:

Time	What I Ate & Drank	How I Feel

Reflections:

Today's physical activity: ....

Today's good habit: ....

♡ **Today I loved my body by:** ....

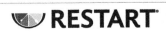

Today is:

Yesterday's bedtime: ___ : ___   Woke up at: ___ : ___   Sleep quality: ___

Water: ☐☐☐☐☐☐☐☐☐☐ (10 oz or 296 ml per box)

BM: ☐ Yes ☐ No   BSC #:

Time	What I Ate & Drank	How I Feel

DAILY JOURNAL

Reflections:

Today's physical activity: ....

Today's good habit: ....

....

♡ **Today I loved my body by:** ....

....

....

....

....

....

....

....

....

....

....

....

....

....

....

....

....

....

....

....

....

....

....

....

....

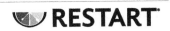

Today is:

Yesterday's bedtime: :   Woke up at: :   Sleep quality:

Water: ☐ ☐ ☐ ☐ ☐ ☐ ☐ ☐ ☐ (10 oz or 296 ml per box)

BM: ☐ Yes   ☐ No   BSC #:

Time	What I Ate & Drank	How I Feel

DAILY JOURNAL

Reflections:

Today's physical activity: ....

Today's good habit: ....

....

♡ **Today I loved my body by:** ....

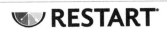

Today is:

Yesterday's bedtime: :   Woke up at: :   Sleep quality:

Water: ☐☐☐☐☐☐☐☐☐☐ (10 oz or 296 ml per box)

BM: ☐ Yes   ☐ No   BSC #:

Time	What I Ate & Drank	How I Feel

Reflections:

Today's physical activity: ....

Today's good habit: ....

♡ **Today I loved my body by:** ....

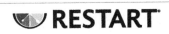

Today is:

Yesterday's bedtime: :   Woke up at: :   Sleep quality:

Water: ☐☐☐☐☐☐☐☐☐ (10 oz or 296 ml per box)

BM: ☐ Yes ☐ No   BSC #:

Time	What I Ate & Drank	How I Feel

Reflections:

Today's physical activity: ....

Today's good habit: ....

....

♡ **Today I loved my body by:** ....

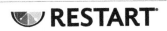

Today is:

Yesterday's bedtime: :   Woke up at: :   Sleep quality:

Water: ☐☐☐☐☐☐☐☐☐ (10 oz or 296 ml per box)

BM: ☐ Yes   ☐ No   BSC #:

Time	What I Ate & Drank	How I Feel

DAILY JOURNAL

Reflections:

Today's physical activity: ....

Today's good habit: ....

♡ **Today I loved my body by:** ....

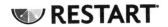

Today is:

Yesterday's bedtime: : Woke up at: : Sleep quality:

Water: ☐ ☐ ☐ ☐ ☐ ☐ ☐ ☐ ☐ (10 oz or 296 ml per box)

BM: ☐ Yes ☐ No BSC #:

Time	What I Ate & Drank	How I Feel

Reflections:

Today's physical activity: ....

Today's good habit: ....

....

♡ **Today I loved my body by:** ....

....

....

....

....

....

....

....

....

....

....

....

....

....

....

....

....

....

....

....

....

....

....

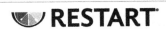

Today is:

Yesterday's bedtime: :   Woke up at: :   Sleep quality:

Water: ☐☐☐☐☐☐☐☐☐☐ (10 oz or 296 ml per box)

BM: ☐ Yes ☐ No   BSC #:

Time	What I Ate & Drank	How I Feel

Reflections:

Today's physical activity: ....

Today's good habit: ....

....

♡ **Today I loved my body by:** ....

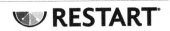

Today is:

Yesterday's bedtime: :   Woke up at: :   Sleep quality:

Water: ☐☐☐☐☐☐☐☐☐ (10 oz or 296 ml per box)

BM: ☐ Yes   ☐ No   BSC #:

Time	What I Ate & Drank	How I Feel

DAILY JOURNAL

Reflections:

Today's physical activity: ....

Today's good habit: ....

♡ **Today I loved my body by:** ....

....

....

....

....

....

....

....

....

....

....

....

....

....

....

....

....

....

....

....

....

....

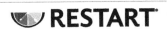

Today is:

Yesterday's bedtime: :   **Woke up at:**   :   **Sleep quality:**

Water: ☐☐☐☐☐☐☐☐☐ (10 oz or 296 ml per box)

BM: ☐ Yes   ☐ No   **BSC #:**

Time	What I Ate & Drank	How I Feel

Reflections:

Today's physical activity: ....

Today's good habit: ....

♡ **Today I loved my body by:** ....

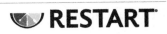

Today is:

Yesterday's bedtime: :   Woke up at: :   Sleep quality:

Water: ☐☐☐☐☐☐☐☐☐ (10 oz or 296 ml per box)

BM: ☐ Yes   ☐ No   BSC #:

Time	What I Ate & Drank	How I Feel

Reflections:

Today's physical activity: ....

Today's good habit: ....

♡ **Today I loved my body by:** ....

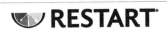

Today is:

Yesterday's bedtime: :   Woke up at: :   Sleep quality:

Water: ☐☐☐☐☐☐☐☐☐☐ (10 oz or 296 ml per box)

BM: ☐ Yes   ☐ No   BSC #:

Time	What I Ate & Drank	How I Feel

Reflections:

Today's physical activity: ....

Today's good habit: ....

♡ **Today I loved my body by:** ....

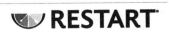

Today is:

Yesterday's bedtime: :   **Woke up at:**   :   **Sleep quality:**

Water: ☐☐☐☐☐☐☐☐☐☐ (10 oz or 296 ml per box)

BM: ☐ Yes   ☐ No   **BSC #:**

Time	What I Ate & Drank	How I Feel

Reflections:

Today's physical activity: ....

Today's good habit: ....

♡ **Today I loved my body by:** ....

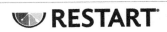

Today is:

Yesterday's bedtime: :   Woke up at: :   Sleep quality:

Water: ☐☐☐☐☐☐☐☐☐ (10 oz or 296 ml per box)

BM: ☐ Yes ☐ No   BSC #:

Time	What I Ate & Drank	How I Feel

Reflections:

Today's physical activity: ....

Today's good habit: ....

♡ **Today I loved my body by:** ....

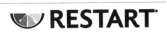

Today is:

Yesterday's bedtime: :   Woke up at: :   Sleep quality:

Water: ☐☐☐☐☐☐☐☐☐ (10 oz or 296 ml per box)

BM: ☐ Yes ☐ No   BSC #:

Time	What I Ate & Drank	How I Feel

Reflections:

Today's physical activity: ....

Today's good habit: ....

♡ **Today I loved my body by:** ....

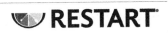

Today is:

Yesterday's bedtime: :   **Woke up at:**   :   **Sleep quality:**

Water: ☐☐☐☐☐☐☐☐☐☐ (10 oz or 296 ml per box)

BM: ☐ Yes   ☐ No   **BSC #:**

Time	What I Ate & Drank	How I Feel

Reflections:

Today's physical activity: ....

Today's good habit: ....

....

♡ Today I loved my body by: ....

....

....

....

....

....

....

....

....

....

....

....

....

....

....

....

....

....

....

....

....

....

....

....

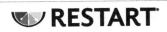

Today is:

Yesterday's bedtime: **:**   Woke up at: **:**   Sleep quality:

Water: ☐☐☐☐☐☐☐☐☐ (10 oz or 296 ml per box)

BM: ☐ Yes ☐ No   BSC #:

Time	What I Ate & Drank	How I Feel

DAILY JOURNAL

Reflections:

Today's physical activity: ....

Today's good habit: ....

♡ **Today I loved my body by:** ....

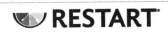

Today is:

Yesterday's bedtime: :   Woke up at: :   Sleep quality:

Water: ☐☐☐☐☐☐☐☐☐☐ (10 oz or 296 ml per box)

BM: ☐ Yes   ☐ No   BSC #:

Time	What I Ate & Drank	How I Feel

DAILY JOURNAL

Reflections:

Today's physical activity: ....

Today's good habit: ....

♡ **Today I loved my body by:** ....

....

....

....

....

....

....

....

....

....

....

....

....

....

....

....

....

....

....

....

....

....

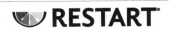 **RESTART**

Today is:

Yesterday's bedtime: :   Woke up at: :   Sleep quality:

Water: ☐☐☐☐☐☐☐☐☐☐ (10 oz or 296 ml per box)

BM: ☐ Yes   ☐ No   BSC #:

Time	What I Ate & Drank	How I Feel

DAILY JOURNAL

Reflections:

Today's physical activity: ....

Today's good habit: ....

♡ **Today I loved my body by:** ....

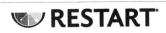

Today is:

Yesterday's bedtime: :   **Woke up at:** :   **Sleep quality:**

Water: ☐☐☐☐☐☐☐☐☐☐ (10 oz or 296 ml per box)

BM: ☐ Yes ☐ No   **BSC #:**

Time	What I Ate & Drank	How I Feel

Reflections:

Today's physical activity: ....

Today's good habit: ....

♡ **Today I loved my body by:** ....

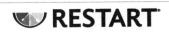

Today is:

Yesterday's bedtime: :   Woke up at: :   Sleep quality:

Water: ☐☐☐☐☐☐☐☐☐ (10 oz or 296 ml per box)

BM: ☐ Yes   ☐ No   BSC #:

Time	What I Ate & Drank	How I Feel

Reflections:

Today's physical activity: ....

Today's good habit: ....

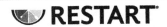 **Today I loved my body by:** ....

Today is:

Yesterday's bedtime: :   Woke up at: :   Sleep quality:

Water: ☐☐☐☐☐☐☐☐☐☐ (10 oz or 296 ml per box)

BM: ☐ Yes   ☐ No   BSC #:

Time	What I Ate & Drank	How I Feel

DAILY JOURNAL

Reflections:

Today's physical activity: ....

Today's good habit: ....

....

♡ **Today I loved my body by:** ....

....

....

....

....

....

....

....

....

....

....

....

....

....

....

....

....

....

....

....

....

....

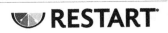

Today is:

Yesterday's bedtime: :   **Woke up at:**   :   **Sleep quality:**

Water: ☐☐☐☐☐☐☐☐☐☐ (10 oz or 296 ml per box)

BM: ☐ Yes   ☐ No   **BSC #:**

Time	What I Ate & Drank	How I Feel

DAILY JOURNAL

Reflections:

Today's physical activity: ....

Today's good habit: ....

♡ **Today I loved my body by:** ....

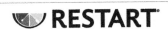

Today is:

Yesterday's bedtime: :   **Woke up at:**   :   **Sleep quality:**

Water: ☐ ☐ ☐ ☐ ☐ ☐ ☐ ☐ ☐ ☐ (10 oz or 296 ml per box)

BM: ☐ Yes   ☐ No   **BSC #:**

Time	What I Ate & Drank	How I Feel

Reflections:

Today's physical activity: ....

Today's good habit: ....

♡ **Today I loved my body by:** ....

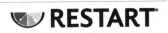

Today is:

Yesterday's bedtime: :   **Woke up at:**   :   **Sleep quality:**

Water: ☐ ☐ ☐ ☐ ☐ ☐ ☐ ☐ ☐ (10 oz or 296 ml per box)

BM: ☐ Yes   ☐ No   **BSC #:**

Time	What I Ate & Drank	How I Feel

DAILY JOURNAL

Reflections:

Today's physical activity: ....

Today's good habit: ....

♡ **Today I loved my body by:** ....

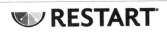

Today is:

Yesterday's bedtime: : Woke up at: : Sleep quality:

Water: ☐☐☐☐☐☐☐☐☐☐ (10 oz or 296 ml per box)

BM: ☐ Yes ☐ No BSC #:

Time	What I Ate & Drank	How I Feel

Reflections:

Today's physical activity: ....

Today's good habit: ....

♡ **Today I loved my body by:** ....

....

....

....

....

....

....

....

....

....

....

....

....

....

....

....

....

....

....

....

....

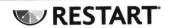

Today is:

Yesterday's bedtime: :   Woke up at: :   Sleep quality:

Water: ☐☐☐☐☐☐☐☐☐☐ (10 oz or 296 ml per box)

BM: ☐ Yes   ☐ No   BSC #:

Time	What I Ate & Drank	How I Feel

DAILY JOURNAL

Reflections:

Today's physical activity: ....

Today's good habit: ....

♡ **Today I loved my body by:** ....

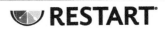

Today is:

Yesterday's bedtime: :   Woke up at: :   Sleep quality:

Water: ☐☐☐☐☐☐☐☐☐☐ (10 oz or 296 ml per box)

BM: ☐ Yes ☐ No   BSC #:

Time	What I Ate & Drank	How I Feel

Reflections:

Today's physical activity: ....

Today's good habit: ....

....

♡ **Today I loved my body by:** ....

....

....

....

....

....

....

....

....

....

....

....

....

....

....

....

....

....

....

....

....

....

....

....

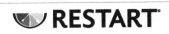

Today is:

Yesterday's bedtime: :   Woke up at: :   Sleep quality:

Water: ☐☐☐☐☐☐☐☐☐☐ (10 oz or 296 ml per box)

BM: ☐ Yes   ☐ No   BSC #:

Time	What I Ate & Drank	How I Feel

Reflections:

Today's physical activity: ....

Today's good habit: ....

....

♡ **Today I loved my body by:** ....

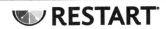

Today is:

Yesterday's bedtime: ___ : ___   **Woke up at:** ___ : ___   **Sleep quality:** ___

Water: ☐☐☐☐☐☐☐☐☐☐ (10 oz or 296 ml per box)

BM: ☐ Yes ☐ No   **BSC #:** ___

Time	What I Ate & Drank	How I Feel

DAILY JOURNAL

Reflections:

Today's physical activity: ....

Today's good habit: ....

....

♡ **Today I loved my body by:** ....

....

....

....

....

....

....

....

....

....

....

....

....

....

....

....

....

....

....

....

....

....

....

....

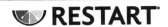

Today is:

Yesterday's bedtime: :   Woke up at: :   Sleep quality:

Water: ☐ ☐ ☐ ☐ ☐ ☐ ☐ ☐ ☐ (10 oz or 296 ml per box)

BM: ☐ Yes ☐ No   BSC #:

Time	What I Ate & Drank	How I Feel

Reflections:

Today's physical activity: ....

Today's good habit: ....

♡ **Today I loved my body by:** ....

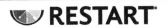

Today is: ....

Yesterday's bedtime: :   **Woke up at:**   :   **Sleep quality:**

Water: ☐☐☐☐☐☐☐☐☐ (10 oz or 296 ml per box)

BM: ☐ Yes   ☐ No   **BSC #:**

Time	What I Ate & Drank	How I Feel

Reflections:

Today's physical activity: ....

Today's good habit: ....

....

♡ **Today I loved my body by:** ....

....

....

....

....

....

....

....

....

....

....

....

....

....

....

....

....

....

....

....

....

....

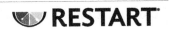

Today is:

Yesterday's bedtime: :   **Woke up at:**   :   **Sleep quality:**

Water: ☐☐☐☐☐☐☐☐☐☐ (10 oz or 296 ml per box)

BM: ☐ Yes   ☐ No   **BSC #:**

Time	What I Ate & Drank	How I Feel

Reflections:

Today's physical activity: ....

Today's good habit: ....

♡ **Today I loved my body by:** ....

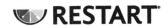

Today is:

Yesterday's bedtime: :   **Woke up at:**   :   **Sleep quality:**

Water: ☐☐☐☐☐☐☐☐☐☐ (10 oz or 296 ml per box)

BM: ☐ Yes   ☐ No   **BSC #:**

Time	What I Ate & Drank	How I Feel

DAILY JOURNAL

Reflections:

Today's physical activity: ....

Today's good habit: ....

♡ **Today I loved my body by:** ....

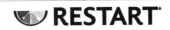

Today is:

Yesterday's bedtime: : Woke up at: : Sleep quality:

Water: ☐☐☐☐☐☐☐☐☐☐ (10 oz or 296 ml per box)

BM: ☐ Yes ☐ No BSC #:

Time	What I Ate & Drank	How I Feel

Reflections:

Today's physical activity: ....

Today's good habit: ....

♡**Today I loved my body by:** ....

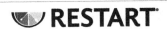

Today is:

Yesterday's bedtime: :   **Woke up at:**   :   **Sleep quality:**

Water: ☐☐☐☐☐☐☐☐☐☐ (10 oz or 296 ml per box)

BM: ☐ Yes   ☐ No   **BSC #:**

Time	What I Ate & Drank	How I Feel

Reflections:

Today's physical activity: ....
Today's good habit: ....
....

♡ **Today I loved my body by:** ....

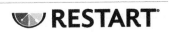

Today is:

Yesterday's bedtime: :   **Woke up at:**   :   **Sleep quality:**

Water: ☐☐☐☐☐☐☐☐☐ (10 oz or 296 ml per box)

BM: ☐ Yes   ☐ No   **BSC #:**

Time	What I Ate & Drank	How I Feel

Reflections:

Today's physical activity: ....

Today's good habit: ....

♡ **Today I loved my body by:** ....

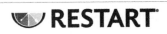

Today is:

Yesterday's bedtime: :   **Woke up at:**   :   **Sleep quality:**

Water: ☐ ☐ ☐ ☐ ☐ ☐ ☐ ☐ ☐ (10 oz or 296 ml per box)

BM: ☐ Yes ☐ No   **BSC #:**

Time	What I Ate & Drank	How I Feel

Reflections:

Today's physical activity: ....

Today's good habit: ....

....

♡ **Today I loved my body by:** ....

....

....

....

....

....

....

....

....

....

....

....

....

....

....

....

....

....

....

....

....

....

....

....

....

....

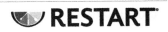

Today is:

Yesterday's bedtime: :   **Woke up at:**   :   **Sleep quality:**

Water: ☐☐☐☐☐☐☐☐☐ (10 oz or 296 ml per box)

BM: ☐ Yes   ☐ No   **BSC #:**

Time	What I Ate & Drank	How I Feel

Reflections:

Today's physical activity: ....

Today's good habit: ....

♡ **Today I loved my body by:** ....

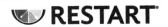

Today is:

Yesterday's bedtime: :   **Woke up at:**   :   **Sleep quality:**

Water: ☐☐☐☐☐☐☐☐☐ (10 oz or 296 ml per box)

BM: ☐ Yes   ☐ No   **BSC #:**

Time	What I Ate & Drank	How I Feel

DAILY JOURNAL

Reflections:

Today's physical activity: ....

Today's good habit: ....

....

♡ **Today I loved my body by:** ....

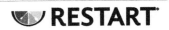

Today is:

Yesterday's bedtime: :   Woke up at: :   Sleep quality:

Water: ☐☐☐☐☐☐☐☐☐ (10 oz or 296 ml per box)

BM: ☐ Yes ☐ No   BSC #:

Time	What I Ate & Drank	How I Feel

DAILY JOURNAL

Reflections:

Today's physical activity: ....

Today's good habit: ....

♡ **Today I loved my body by:** ....

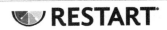

Today is:

Yesterday's bedtime: : **Woke up at:** : **Sleep quality:**

Water: ☐☐☐☐☐☐☐☐☐☐ (10 oz or 296 ml per box)

BM: ☐ Yes ☐ No **BSC #:**

Time	What I Ate & Drank	How I Feel

DAILY JOURNAL

Reflections:

Today's physical activity: ....

Today's good habit: ....

....

♡ **Today I loved my body by:** ....

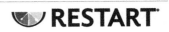

Today is:

Yesterday's bedtime: :   Woke up at: :   Sleep quality:

Water: ☐☐☐☐☐☐☐☐☐ (10 oz or 296 ml per box)

BM: ☐ Yes ☐ No   BSC #:

Time	What I Ate & Drank	How I Feel

DAILY JOURNAL

Reflections:

Today's physical activity: ....

Today's good habit: ....

....

♡ **Today I loved my body by:** ....

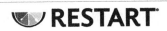

Today is:

Yesterday's bedtime: :   **Woke up at:**   :   **Sleep quality:**

Water: ☐☐☐☐☐☐☐☐☐☐ (10 oz or 296 ml per box)

BM: ☐ Yes ☐ No   **BSC #:**

Time	What I Ate & Drank	How I Feel

Reflections:

Today's physical activity: ....

Today's good habit: ....

♡ **Today I loved my body by:** ....

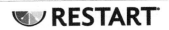

Today is:

Yesterday's bedtime: :   **Woke up at:**   :   **Sleep quality:**

Water: ☐☐☐☐☐☐☐☐☐☐ (10 oz or 296 ml per box)

BM: ☐ Yes   ☐ No   **BSC #:**

Time	What I Ate & Drank	How I Feel

Reflections:

Today's physical activity: ....

Today's good habit: ....

♡ **Today I loved my body by:** ....

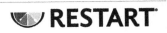

Today is:

Yesterday's bedtime: :   Woke up at: :   Sleep quality:

Water: ☐☐☐☐☐☐☐☐☐ (10 oz or 296 ml per box)

BM: ☐ Yes   ☐ No   BSC #:

Time	What I Ate & Drank	How I Feel

DAILY JOURNAL

Reflections:

Today's physical activity: ....

Today's good habit: ....

....

♡ **Today I loved my body by:** ....

....

....

....

....

....

....

....

....

....

....

....

....

....

....

....

....

....

....

....

....

....

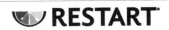

Today is:

Yesterday's bedtime: :   **Woke up at:**   :   **Sleep quality:**

Water: ☐☐☐☐☐☐☐☐☐☐ (10 oz or 296 ml per box)

BM: ☐ Yes   ☐ No   **BSC #:**

Time	What I Ate & Drank	How I Feel

DAILY JOURNAL

Reflections:

Today's physical activity: ....

Today's good habit: ....

♡ **Today I loved my body by:** ....

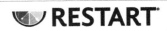

Today is:

Yesterday's bedtime: ⠀⠀:⠀⠀ **Woke up at:** ⠀⠀:⠀⠀ **Sleep quality:**

Water: ☐☐☐☐☐☐☐☐☐ (10 oz or 296 ml per box)

BM: ☐ Yes ☐ No ⠀ **BSC #:**

Time	What I Ate & Drank	How I Feel

DAILY JOURNAL

Reflections:

Today's physical activity: ....

Today's good habit: ....

♡ **Today I loved my body by:** ....

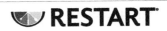

Today is:

Yesterday's bedtime: : **Woke up at:** : **Sleep quality:**

Water: ☐☐☐☐☐☐☐☐☐ (10 oz or 296 ml per box)

BM: ☐ Yes ☐ No **BSC #:**

Time	What I Ate & Drank	How I Feel

Reflections:

Today's physical activity: ....

Today's good habit: ....

♡ **Today I loved my body by:** ....

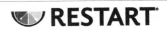

Today is:

Yesterday's bedtime: :   Woke up at: :   Sleep quality:

Water: ☐☐☐☐☐☐☐☐☐ (10 oz or 296 ml per box)

BM: ☐ Yes   ☐ No   BSC #:

Time	What I Ate & Drank	How I Feel

DAILY JOURNAL

Reflections:

Today's physical activity: ....

Today's good habit: ....

....

♡ **Today I loved my body by:** ....

....

....

....

....

....

....

....

....

....

....

....

....

....

....

....

....

....

....

....

....

....

....

....

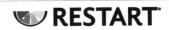

Today is:

Yesterday's bedtime: : Woke up at: : Sleep quality:

Water: ☐☐☐☐☐☐☐☐☐☐ (10 oz or 296 ml per box)

BM: ☐ Yes ☐ No BSC #:

Time	What I Ate & Drank	How I Feel

DAILY JOURNAL

Reflections:

Today's physical activity: ....

Today's good habit: ....

♡ **Today I loved my body by:** ....

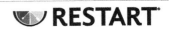

Today is:

Yesterday's bedtime: ⠀ : ⠀⠀ **Woke up at:** ⠀ : ⠀⠀ **Sleep quality:**

Water: ☐☐☐☐☐☐☐☐☐ (10 oz or 296 ml per box)

BM: ☐ Yes ☐ No ⠀ **BSC #:**

Time	What I Ate & Drank	How I Feel

Reflections:

Today's physical activity: ....

Today's good habit: ....

....

♡ **Today I loved my body by:** ....

....

....

....

....

....

....

....

....

....

....

....

....

....

....

....

....

....

....

....

....

....

....

....

....

....

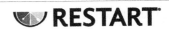

Today is:

Yesterday's bedtime: **:**   Woke up at: **:**   Sleep quality:

Water: ☐☐☐☐☐☐☐☐☐☐ (10 oz or 296 ml per box)

BM: ☐ Yes ☐ No   BSC #:

Time	What I Ate & Drank	How I Feel

Reflections:

Today's physical activity: ....

Today's good habit: ....

♡ **Today I loved my body by:** ....

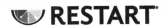

Today is:

Yesterday's bedtime: :   **Woke up at:**   :   **Sleep quality:**

Water: ☐☐☐☐☐☐☐☐☐☐ (10 oz or 296 ml per box)

BM: ☐ Yes   ☐ No   **BSC #:**

Time	What I Ate & Drank	How I Feel

Reflections:

Today's physical activity: ....

Today's good habit: ....

....

♡ **Today I loved my body by:** ....

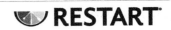

Today is:

Yesterday's bedtime: :   Woke up at: :   Sleep quality:

Water: ☐☐☐☐☐☐☐☐☐☐ (10 oz or 296 ml per box)

BM: ☐ Yes   ☐ No   BSC #:

Time	What I Ate & Drank	How I Feel

Reflections:

Today's physical activity: ....

Today's good habit: ....

♡**Today I loved my body by:** ....

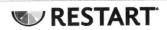

Today is:

Yesterday's bedtime: :   **Woke up at:**   :   **Sleep quality:**

Water: ☐☐☐☐☐☐☐☐☐ (10 oz or 296 ml per box)

BM: ☐ Yes   ☐ No   **BSC #:**

Time	What I Ate & Drank	How I Feel

Reflections:

Today's physical activity: ....

Today's good habit: ....

....

♡ **Today I loved my body by:** ....

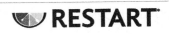

Today is:

Yesterday's bedtime: :   Woke up at: :   Sleep quality:

Water: ☐☐☐☐☐☐☐☐☐☐ (10 oz or 296 ml per box)

BM: ☐ Yes ☐ No   BSC #:

Time	What I Ate & Drank	How I Feel

Reflections:

Today's physical activity: ....

Today's good habit: ....

♡ **Today I loved my body by:** ....

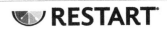

Today is:

Yesterday's bedtime: :   **Woke up at:**   :   **Sleep quality:**

Water: ☐☐☐☐☐☐☐☐☐☐ (10 oz or 296 ml per box)

BM: ☐ Yes ☐ No   **BSC #:**

Time	What I Ate & Drank	How I Feel

Reflections:

Today's physical activity: ....

Today's good habit: ....

....

♡ **Today I loved my body by:** ....

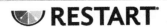

Today is:

Yesterday's bedtime: :   Woke up at: :   Sleep quality:

Water: ☐☐☐☐☐☐☐☐☐☐ (10 oz or 296 ml per box)

BM: ☐ Yes ☐ No   BSC #:

Time	What I Ate & Drank	How I Feel

DAILY JOURNAL

Reflections:

Today's physical activity: ....

Today's good habit: ....

♡ **Today I loved my body by:** ....

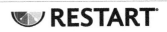

Today is:

Yesterday's bedtime: ___ : ___   Woke up at: ___ : ___   Sleep quality: ___

Water: ☐☐☐☐☐☐☐☐☐ (10 oz or 296 ml per box)

BM: ☐ Yes   ☐ No   BSC #:

Time	What I Ate & Drank	How I Feel

DAILY JOURNAL

Reflections:

Today's physical activity: ....

Today's good habit: ....

....

♡ **Today I loved my body by:** ....

....
....
....
....
....
....
....
....
....
....
....
....
....
....
....
....
....
....
....
....
....
....
....
....
....
....
....

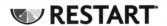

Today is:

Yesterday's bedtime: :   Woke up at: :   Sleep quality:

Water: ☐☐☐☐☐☐☐☐☐☐ (10 oz or 296 ml per box)

BM: ☐ Yes ☐ No   BSC #:

Time	What I Ate & Drank	How I Feel

Reflections:

Today's physical activity: ....
Today's good habit: ....

♡ **Today I loved my body by:** ....

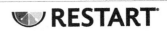

Today is:

Yesterday's bedtime: :   **Woke up at:** :   **Sleep quality:**

Water: ☐☐☐☐☐☐☐☐☐☐ (10 oz or 296 ml per box)

BM: ☐ Yes ☐ No   **BSC #:**

Time	What I Ate & Drank	How I Feel

Reflections:

Today's physical activity: ....

Today's good habit: ....

....

♡ **Today I loved my body by:** ....

....

....

....

....

....

....

....

....

....

....

....

....

....

....

....

....

....

....

....

....

....

....

....

....

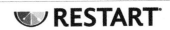

Today is:

Yesterday's bedtime: :   Woke up at: :   Sleep quality:

Water: ☐☐☐☐☐☐☐☐☐☐ (10 oz or 296 ml per box)

BM: ☐ Yes   ☐ No   BSC #:

Time	What I Ate & Drank	How I Feel

DAILY JOURNAL

Reflections:

Today's physical activity: ....

Today's good habit: ....

....

♡ **Today I loved my body by:** ....

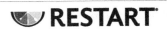

Today is:

Yesterday's bedtime: ____ : ____   Woke up at: ____ : ____   Sleep quality: ____

Water: ☐☐☐☐☐☐☐☐☐☐ (10 oz or 296 ml per box)

BM: ☐ Yes ☐ No   BSC #: ____

Time	What I Ate & Drank	How I Feel

Reflections:

Today's physical activity: ....

Today's good habit: ....

♡ **Today I loved my body by:** ....

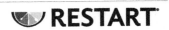

Today is: ....

Yesterday's bedtime: :   **Woke up at:**   :   **Sleep quality:**

Water: ☐☐☐☐☐☐☐☐☐☐ (10 oz or 296 ml per box)

BM: ☐ Yes   ☐ No   **BSC #:**

Time	What I Ate & Drank	How I Feel

DAILY JOURNAL

Reflections:

Today's physical activity: ....

Today's good habit: ....

♡ **Today I loved my body by:** ....

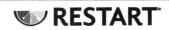

Today is: ....

Yesterday's bedtime: :   **Woke up at:**   :   **Sleep quality:**

Water: ☐☐☐☐☐☐☐☐☐☐ (10 oz or 296 ml per box)

BM: ☐ Yes ☐ No   **BSC #:**

Time	What I Ate & Drank	How I Feel

Reflections:

Today's physical activity: ....

Today's good habit: ....

....

♡ **Today I loved my body by:** ....

....

....

....

....

....

....

....

....

....

....

....

....

....

....

....

....

....

....

....

....

....

....

....

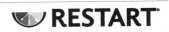

Today is:

Yesterday's bedtime: :   **Woke up at:**   :   **Sleep quality:**

Water: ☐☐☐☐☐☐☐☐☐☐ (10 oz or 296 ml per box)

BM: ☐ Yes   ☐ No   **BSC #:**

Time	What I Ate & Drank	How I Feel

Reflections:

Today's physical activity: ....

Today's good habit: ....

♡**Today I loved my body by:** ....

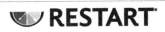

Today is:

Yesterday's bedtime: ___ : ___ **Woke up at:** ___ : ___ **Sleep quality:** ___

Water: ☐☐☐☐☐☐☐☐☐☐ (10 oz or 296 ml per box)

BM: ☐ Yes ☐ No **BSC #:** ___

Time	What I Ate & Drank	How I Feel

DAILY JOURNAL

Reflections:

Today's physical activity: ....

Today's good habit: ....

....

♡ **Today I loved my body by:** ....

....

....

....

....

....

....

....

....

....

....

....

....

....

....

....

....

....

....

....

....

....

....

....

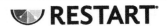

Today is:

Yesterday's bedtime: : Woke up at: : Sleep quality:

Water: ☐☐☐☐☐☐☐☐☐☐ (10 oz or 296 ml per box)

BM: ☐ Yes ☐ No BSC #:

Time	What I Ate & Drank	How I Feel

Reflections:

Today's physical activity: ....

Today's good habit: ....

....

♡ **Today I loved my body by:** ....

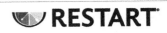

Today is: ....

Yesterday's bedtime:　：　　**Woke up at:**　：　　**Sleep quality:**

Water: ☐☐☐☐☐☐☐☐☐☐ (10 oz or 296 ml per box)

BM: ☐ Yes　☐ No　**BSC #:**

Time	What I Ate & Drank	How I Feel

Reflections:

Today's physical activity: ....

Today's good habit: ....

....

♡ **Today I loved my body by:** ....

....
....
....
....
....
....
....
....
....
....
....
....
....
....
....
....
....
....
....
....
....
....
....

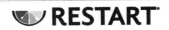 **RESTART**

Today is:
....

Yesterday's bedtime: :   **Woke up at:**   :   **Sleep quality:**

Water: ☐☐☐☐☐☐☐☐☐☐ (10 oz or 296 ml per box)

BM: ☐ Yes   ☐ No   **BSC #:**

Time	What I Ate & Drank	How I Feel

DAILY JOURNAL

Reflections:

Today's physical activity: ....

Today's good habit: ....

♡ **Today I loved my body by:** ....

....

....

....

....

....

....

....

....

....

....

....

....

....

....

....

....

....

....

....

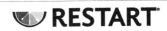

Today is:

Yesterday's bedtime: :   Woke up at: :   Sleep quality:

Water: ☐☐☐☐☐☐☐☐☐☐ (10 oz or 296 ml per box)

BM: ☐ Yes   ☐ No   BSC #:

Time	What I Ate & Drank	How I Feel

Reflections:

Today's physical activity: ....

Today's good habit: ....

....

♡ **Today I loved my body by:** ....

....

....

....

....

....

....

....

....

....

....

....

....

....

....

....

....

....

....

....

....

....

....

....

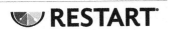

Today is:

Yesterday's bedtime: :   **Woke up at:**   :   **Sleep quality:**

Water: ☐☐☐☐☐☐☐☐☐☐ (10 oz or 296 ml per box)

BM: ☐ Yes   ☐ No   **BSC #:**

Time	What I Ate & Drank	How I Feel

Reflections:

Today's physical activity: ....

Today's good habit: ....

♡ **Today I loved my body by:** ....

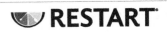

Today is:

Yesterday's bedtime: :   Woke up at: :   Sleep quality:

Water: ☐☐☐☐☐☐☐☐☐ (10 oz or 296 ml per box)

BM: ☐ Yes   ☐ No   BSC #:

Time	What I Ate & Drank	How I Feel

DAILY JOURNAL

Reflections:

Today's physical activity: ....

Today's good habit: ....

....

♡ **Today I loved my body by:** ....

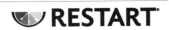

Today is:

Yesterday's bedtime: :   **Woke up at:**   :   **Sleep quality:**

Water: ☐☐☐☐☐☐☐☐☐☐ (10 oz or 296 ml per box)

BM: ☐ Yes   ☐ No   **BSC #:**

Time	What I Ate & Drank	How I Feel

Reflections:

Today's physical activity: ....

Today's good habit: ....

♡ **Today I loved my body by:** ....

....

....

....

....

....

....

....

....

....

....

....

....

....

....

....

....

....

....

....

....

....

....

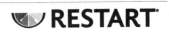

Today is:

Yesterday's bedtime: : **Woke up at:** : **Sleep quality:**

Water: ☐☐☐☐☐☐☐☐☐☐ (10 oz or 296 ml per box)

BM: ☐ Yes ☐ No **BSC #:**

Time	What I Ate & Drank	How I Feel

Reflections:

Today's physical activity: ....

Today's good habit: ....

♡ **Today I loved my body by:** ....

....

....

....

....

....

....

....

....

....

....

....

....

....

....

....

....

....

....

....

....

....

....

....

....

....

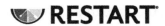

Today is:

Yesterday's bedtime: :   Woke up at: :   Sleep quality:

Water: ☐☐☐☐☐☐☐☐☐☐ (10 oz or 296 ml per box)

BM: ☐ Yes   ☐ No   BSC #:

Time	What I Ate & Drank	How I Feel

Reflections:

Today's physical activity: ....

Today's good habit: ....

♡ **Today I loved my body by:** ....

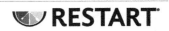

Today is: ....

Yesterday's bedtime: :   **Woke up at:**   :   **Sleep quality:**

Water: ☐☐☐☐☐☐☐☐☐☐ (10 oz or 296 ml per box)

BM: ☐ Yes   ☐ No   **BSC #:**

Time	What I Ate & Drank	How I Feel

Reflections:

Today's physical activity: ....

Today's good habit: ....

....

♡ **Today I loved my body by:** ....

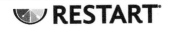

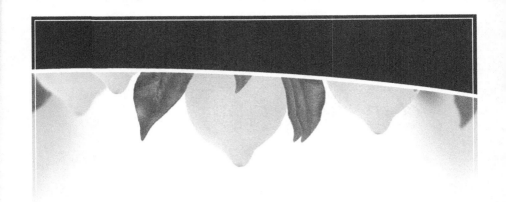

get in the...

HABIT

"Today's good habit" – What healthful habit(s) are you working on? You can work on the same habit each day until you have mastered it, or you can work on something new each week to keep the challenge fresh. Use this handy chart to help you track your progress.

Get in the habit...

	1	2	3	4	5	6	7	8	9	10	11	12
HABIT 1:												
HABIT 2:												
HABIT 3:												
HABIT 4:												
HABIT 5:												
HABIT 6:												
HABIT 7:												
HABIT 8:												
HABIT 9:												
HABIT 10:												
HABIT 11:												
HABIT 12:												

13	14	15	16	17	18	19	20	21	22	23	24	25	26	27	28	29	30	31

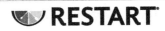

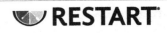

Ready to learn more?

 GET INSPIRED

For recipes, learning and support, visit us at our website and on social media.

Visit our website at **www.TheRestartProgram.com**

on Facebook at: **www.facebook.com/TheRestartProgram**

on Pinterest at: **www.pinterest.com/therestartprog/**

on Instagram: **www.instagram.com/therestartprogram/**

A perfect companion to your real food experience:
The RESTART® Cookbook

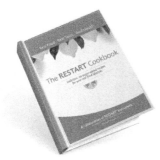

Enjoy this compilation of recipes from RESTART® Instructors. Prepare delicious, no added sugar recipes for every meal.

Order yours on Amazon today!

Made in the USA
Monee, IL
05 September 2022

13293546R00111